THE RIDICULOUSLY SIMPLE GUIDE TO BABY FIRST AID AND COMMON ILLNESSES

A PRACTICAL GUIDE FOR NEW PARENTS

MARGO JEAN

Ridiculously Simple Press
ANAHEIM, CALIFORNIA

Contents

i

Disclaimer: this book is meant to be a quick reference to help you understand what's going on with your baby and what you can do about it. *This book is not meant to replace or ignore medical advice.*

INTRODUCTION

HAVING A BABY IS scary! Like you might as well sleep with one eye open scary! It feels like a million things can go wrong. The Internet doesn't help things—no, Mom, I have not read the story of the baby who choked on their fingernail, but thanks for giving one more thing to worry about!

This book isn't a guide to solving everything that could go wrong. It's a easy and quick reference to the most common things and how to treat them.

The first section covers first aid. The second section is the most common illnesses.

Babies can suffer many different ailments in the first few years of life. Most of them are common and easily treatable. It is important, however, to know when and how to treat, and when to see a doctor. The list below are several common topics of Infant First Aid.

[1]

Baby First Aid

MANY OF THE TOPICS covered in this first section are best treated with CPR. The below section is meant to help you understand Baby CPR, but should not be used in lieu of it. Baby CPR is something all parents should learn, and there are plenty of trainings available (some free) in cities across the United States. Check with your local hospital for referrals.

Baby CPR

Cardiopulmonary Resuscitation, or better known as CPR is something that every parent should be familiar with. Infant CPR is a little bit different than the adult version of a series of chest compressions and breathing. You would of course, first check to see if the baby is breathing, but instead of full fist compressions, you would use two fingers instead.

In the very unfortunate event that you ever need to help revive your baby, you may have to use baby CPR. The most crucial moments are the first couple of minutes once baby stops breathing. It is a very good idea to take a professional course, most only last a couple of hours, and could save your baby's life in an emergency.

To engage in CPR, you would follow certain procedures. First, and most important, call 911. Next, check and clear the airway if necessary, and then you would complete a series of 10 chest compressions with your first two fingers only. Try to compress down about a half inch, but no more. Then breath into baby's mouth, making sure nose is blocked. If necessary, cover both mouth and nose with your mouth to complete breaths. Repeat these steps until help arrives or baby starts breathing on his own.

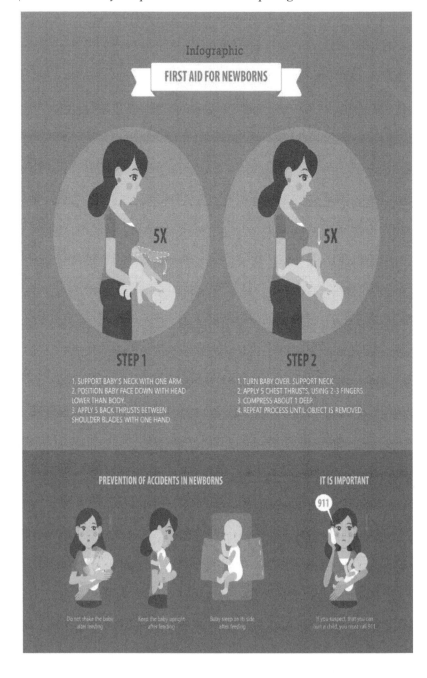

CHOKING BABY

When a baby's airway becomes blocked, they may begin to choke. This can happen while eating, but it may also happen at different times. Food or toys of all different sizes could get caught in baby's mouth or throat. If an object becomes lodged in an infant's airway, they may be unable to breath and suffocation can occur.

How to Treat

Choking is something that all parents should be able to effectively treat. Besides not having the development to chew and swallow everything properly, one of the primary ways babies learn about their environment is putting everything in their mouths. One of the most practiced forms of dislodging an item from a baby's airway is the Heimlich Maneuver. First, give the baby five chest thrusts. Using your first two fingers, compress the baby's chest about a half an inch deep. Then, flip baby onto his stomach, use your knee for support to put baby on a downward angle and slap baby's back 5 times. Repeat these steps until the object comes out.

When to see a doctor

As soon as you fear that baby is choking, call 911. The operator can guide you through the process of practicing the Heimlich Maneuver on baby and send help if needed.

SEVERE BLEEDING

Severe bleeding is exactly what it sounds like, blood flow that does not stop. This could be from an abrasion or wound and should be treated immediately.

How to Treat

The first thing that you should do if your baby is suffering from severe bleeding is assess the situation. Is the baby conscious? Where is the blood coming from? If the baby seems to be going into shock, get help right away. Lay baby down and raise his feet to help get blood flow to the brain. Then find the wound, and with a bandage or cloth, put pressure on the wound to try and stop the bleeding. Continue to add layers of bandages if needed, and use plastic wrap to loosely, but securely, keep the bandage in place.

When to see a doctor

If your baby is bleeding severely, it is an emergency. Call, or have someone call 911 immediately if your baby is unresponsive. If baby is alert, once you control the bleeding seek medical attention as soon as possible.

CUTS/ABRASIONS

Cuts and abrasions are inevitable with little ones. Their curiosity often overrides their knowledge of their surroundings and accidents often happen. A cut or abrasion would be when your little one has an open wound, but it is not bleeding uncontrollably.

How to Treat

As with any other wound, the first thing that you should do is assess the situation. Try to find out what caused the cut or abrasion and make sure that it wasn't something extremely toxic. Since babies can't talk, this might be difficult, but look around for anything sharp or dangerous and be sure to remove it from the environment. Then you should thoroughly clean the area with a gentle antiseptic or warm soap and water to prevent infection. If the abrasion is large or deep enough, cover the wound with a bandage until it clots completely.

When to See a Doctor

If you can control the bleeding of the abrasion and it doesn't look too deep there is no real need to get medical attention unless you are worried that the cause of the abrasion could be harmful. Call a doctor if swelling or severe redness occurs, or if you notice signs of infection.

INFECTED WOUNDS

An infected wound is one that shows no sign of healing. It may be red around the edges, swollen or have cloudy, white, or green pus seeping from the abrasion. If you notice that your baby is extremely sensitive in that area there is probably tenderness or pain, which is another sign of infection.

How to Treat

Germs are everywhere, so it is common that open wounds may become infected. If you notice signs of infection, you should keep the wound extra clean, but also get to the doctor right away. You do not want the infection to travel further away from the wound and complicate your baby's immune system. Use a cold compress, like a washcloth, to ease discomfort temporarily. Keep the wound covered and clean until you receive further directions from a medical professional.

When to see a doctor

It is pretty important to take baby to see a doctor at the first signs of an infected wound. The longer you wait, the more damage that can be done.

BLISTERS

Blisters are little bumps on your baby's skin that are filled with fluid. Blisters can be caused by a number of different things such as sunburn, bug bites, and contact dermatitis. Some viruses and bacterial infections may also cause blisters to form.

How to Treat

Blisters are typically simple to treat, because there is really nothing you can do except wait it out. If you notice a blister on your baby, try to figure out the cause. If it is from clothing or shoes that are too tight, remove the source and put a small bandage on it. Let your baby go barefoot for a couple of days. Blisters usually heal by themselves. However, if there is a different cause for blisters such as a sickness or burn, you should probably seek medical attention right away. If you have already seen a doctor and your baby has been diagnosed with a sickness, call the doctor to ensure that the blisters are a typical side effect of the illness.

When to call a doctor

It is time to take baby to the doctor if the blister shows signs of infection. If you notice extreme redness and swelling, or baby is ultra sensitive to the touch, you should make an appointment right away. If blisters show up in numbers unexpectedly, it is a good idea to get medical advice on how to treat baby.

NOSE BLEEDS

Nose bleeds can be scary, but they are pretty common, even in infants. Blood will seep out of the nostrils for a number of different reasons. One is simply that the nose is irritated or scratched. A bump on the nose or slight trauma can also cause the nose to bleed. Sometimes even the strain from trying to release a bowel movement will be enough for your infant to get a nose bleed.

How to treat

If your baby does get a nose bleed, try not to get alarmed. There is not enough blood loss from a nose bleed to cause any major damage to your baby. With your baby's head titled slightly forward, apply pressure to the soft sides of the nose with your thumb and index finger using a tissue or soft wash cloth. Do this for about 10 minutes. If this does not stop the bleeding, you can repeat this step for an additional 10 minutes. Using a cold compress on the bridge of the nose can help assist in stopping bleeding, and you can also plug the nostril with gauze.

When to call a doctor

You should bring baby to the doctor immediately if the nose bleed was cause by a severe blow to the nose, just in case. It is also a good idea to seek medical attention if the bleeding does not stop after several hours. If you notice bleeding in other areas of the child at the same time or it is accompanied by a high fever, you should make an appointment to see you doctor.

EAR WOUND

An ear wound is an injury to the ear. Since the ear has both internal and external features wounds can sometimes be hard to identify, especially when your infant is incapable of explaining pain. External ear wounds are visible; they may be in the form of a cut or scratch. Internal wounds could be caused by blunt trauma, an object entering the ear canal, or an infection.

How to Treat

Treatment for the ear depends on the type of wound. If the ear is simply scraped or bruised, clean the area with soap and water and use a dab of antibiotic ointment to prevent infection. Continue to clean area and apply ointment until the wound is healed. These types of wounds generally heal in 2-3 days. If you suspect the ear wound is internal, you should only treat for pain. Give your child acetaminophen as per dosage suggestion and call a doctor to get further advice. A warm cloth or compress may help ease the pain as well.

When to call a doctor

If your child's equilibrium seems to be off, or you feel hearing has been effected it is a good idea to go to the ER. You should also seek immediate medical attention if you see blood or clear liquid oozing out of the ear or you know that an object was entered into the ear canal. For external wounds, go to the doctor if you feel that it is large enough for stitches. However, if there is minimal blood coming from the ear, you can call your doctor and get advice on whether or not to go in. However, if your child is under a year old, any ear wound should get medical attention just to be sure everything is okay.

MOUTH WOUND

Through exploration, play, and just simply being a baby, little ones tend to find themselves with a boo boo on the mouth. Swollen lips from little bangs, bumped gums or teeth, cuts from objects, and cracked lips are pretty common among those in the baby world.

How to Treat

Sometimes mouth injuries are a lot worse than they seem. Gums tend to bleed a lot and the sight of that blood can be alarming, especially to a new parent. Try to stay calm, this will help baby feel better faster and allow you to treat the wound effectively. Use a cool washcloth to clean the area and try to see exactly what the wound it. Try to stop the bleeding if there is any by providing a little pressure with a cool cloth, and provide pain relief as needed with a cold compress or baby pain medicine. Be gentle with feedings and cleaning over the next couple of days, and just keep an eye out for swelling and infection.

> ### When to call a doctor
>
> *Call your doctor if there is bleeding that won't stop after 10 minutes. If the wound is larger than a half inch and severely bleeding, it is a good idea to seek medical attention. Since a lot of mouth wounds are a result from falling, you should go to the doctor if the wound is very dirty or caused by a dirty object. If you begin to see signs of infection like redness, pus or swelling around the edges of the wound, seek medical attention right away. Go to the ER if there is a puncture wound on the roof of the mouth or back of the throat, or if the wound was caused by an animal or human bite.*

BURNS

There are three levels of burns that can be caused from a number of hazards.

First degree burns are the least dangerous and you will most likely just see redness as a result. Second degree burns are more serious and blisters will form where the burn took place. The most severe are third degree burns, and these burns will often appear white, brown or charred and can cause nerve damage.

How to Treat

For all types of burns, the first thing that you should do is to remove the heat source. Get your child away from what is causing the burn. For first degree burns, run the area under cold water and apply aloe to the area. For second and third degree burns, call emergency services, i.e. 911. While you are waiting for help, lie your child down and remove clothing from the area. Elevate the burned area. You can apply cold water or compresses, but be very careful as skin can be super sensitive. Administer acetaminophen for pain relief.

When to call a doctor

Burns are pretty serious, and more often than not they should be treated by a medical professional. You should go see your doctor and time your child is injured from fire or an electrical device, or if it is on his face, genital area, head, or hands. If you think baby has a second or third-degree burn, go right to the ER. If you feel that the burn is covering more than 10% of baby's body call 911 immediately.

SWALLOWED CHEMICAL

If your baby accidentally gets his hands on a bottle of cleaner, nail polish remover, or any other chemical, his first response might be to put it in his mouth. When he does, it is a possibility that he may swallow some of the chemicals inside, obviously, this is dangerous and could cause some medical problems.

How to Treat

The first thing you should do is take the chemical away from baby. Get any poison residue out of the mouth by trying to get baby to spit it out. Make sure to keep a sample of the chemical to determine its dangers once you get medical assistance. Unlike what might seem like a natural response, do not try to make your child throw up. Whatever went down could be just as dangerous coming back up. Have the number to poison control on hand, and call them right away. If you think that you need immediate medical help call 911.

When to call a doctor

Call 911 if you notice that your baby is drowsy, is unconscious, has trouble breathing, is dizzy, or is complaining of severe throat pain. Otherwise, if you feel that there was little to no ingestion, call poison control or your doctor's office and follow their advice and what precautions to take.

SWALLOWED DRUG/ALCOHOL

In the unfortunate event that a little one gets his hands on over-the-counter or prescription medicines or alcohol, and he swallows them, the possibility of poisoning can occur.

How to Treat

The only way to treat the ingestion of any type of drug or alcohol ingestion with your little one is to call 911 or get right to the emergency. Many types of prescription or over the counter medications can be extremely harmful, and should be assessed by a medical professional immediately. Do not try to self-assess and treat, get a professional to handle this one. Try to keep baby comfortable and awake until help arrives. And try to stay calm yourself. Be sure to bring whatever it is that baby ingested so that they can be treated correctly.

When to call a doctor

If your baby accidentally ingests drugs or alcohol, do not wait, get to the ER as soon as possible.

ATE PLANT

There are some household plants that could be poisonous for baby. Ingesting as little as one leaf can cause symptoms to occur. However, even if the plant is not poisonous, eating a plant could be a choking hazard or cause an allergic reaction.

How to Treat

If you notice that your child is getting a reaction to anything, first thing you should do is make an appointment with your doctor. If you feel that the reaction is severe, go to the emergency room or call 911. Make sure to remove and leftover pieces of plant from your child's mouth and give them small sips of water. Do not try to get baby to throw up as it can cause more damage. If the plant was non-poisonous you will probably see little to no reaction. Just keep an eye on baby and call a doctor if you notice anything out of the ordinary such as vomiting or fainting.

When to call a doctor

If you are unfamiliar with the danger of the type of plant your child ingested, call poison control, they will be able to help you. Take your child to a doctor if you notice any symptoms that may indicate poisoning such as rash, difficulty breathing, excessive diarrhea or vomiting, loss of consciousness or heart palpitations. Bring a clipping of the plant with you so doctors can determine its level of toxicity.

FOREIGN OBJECT IN EYE

Sometimes a little something can get stuck in baby's' eye. A piece of dust, a small piece of food, or maybe a little bug. More uncommonly, a larger object, like a toy, may get into babies' eye and this would call for immediate medical attention.

How to treat?

If baby gets a foreign object in his eye, try to remove it first by blowing a little bit. If it does not come out, use an eye wash to try and flush the object out. Do not stick your fingers in baby's eye as it can cause further damage and scratch the eye's cornea. If your baby tries to use his own hands or fingers to try and remove the object, hold his hands and distract him. Try to get him to keep blinking instead in order to remove the object from the eye.

When to call a doctor

If your baby gets an object lodged in his eye, take him to the doctor if it looks like he may have scratched the cornea. Also be alarmed if you start to see signs of infection, redness, excretion of pus, or crust forming around the edges. Seek immediate attention if you see blood coming from the eye or if the object was dirty or rusty and lacerated the cornea or skin around the eye.

FOREIGN OBJECT IN NOSE

Sometimes things end up in the weirdest places, the nose being one of them. Small children like to experiment with finding places for things, but sometimes that doesn't work out so well. An older sibling may think that baby's nose is a good hiding place for their cereal o's, but they will soon find out that it's not that easy to retrieve that snack. Toys and other small objects can also find their way into a nostril, and getting it out might take a little bit of work.

How to Treat

Be careful with trying to remove it yourself as you can accidentally cause it to go further up the nostril. Using tweezers or other tools can actually cause more harm as they can scratch the nose while in use. If your child is old enough to follow directions, see if you can hold the unaffected nostril closed and have him blow until he dislodges the object from his nose. You can also try to blow it out yourself if your child is unable to do so himself. Cover the child's nostril with your fingers and gently blow into the child's mouth to try and dislodge the object.

> **When to call a doctor**
>
> *Seek medical attention if the object is not visibly or easily retrievable. It might seem silly, but go to the doctor if you cannot get the object out with your fingers.*

FOREIGN OBJECT IN EAR

The ear cavity is just large enough for little objects to get through. Sometimes things will end up in there on their own, but other times and object could mistakenly or experimentally placed inside the ear canal. A curious child may think that the ear is a good place to hide something, when in actuality, it's not a good place at all.

How to Treat

If the object is visible and you can easily remove it, then do so. However, do not try and remove something that may move away from you. Sticking things into your child's ear in an attempt to remove an object may in turn make it worse so it is probably best to leave it alone and take your child to see a medical professional. Try to keep your child from sticking his own fingers in his ear to try and remove the object. If possible, hold your child's hands and just reassure him that everything is going to be alright.

> ### *When to call a doctor*
>
> *Call the doctor if the object is not visible. If you can see that there is something in the ear, but you are unsure that you can get it out safely, wait for a professional to do it for you. You could accidentally cause more harm trying to remove the object yourself.*

INSECT BITE

Insect bites are inevitable, especially in the summertime. Baby can get bit by mosquitoes, bees, spiders, or even gnats. An insect bite may show some swelling on baby's skin, unless they have an allergic reaction, which would cause severe swelling, or worse.

How to Treat

Most insect bites do not require treatment, but rather methods to make your child more comfortable. If you notice that your baby has small bumps that resemble mosquito or another small insect bite you can ease their discomfort with a cool cloth or a dab paste made from baking soda and water. If your baby is over six months old, topical hydrocortisone cream may be applied, but it is best to get a recommendation from your pediatrician first. For larger insect bites like bees or wasps, wrap an ice cube in a cloth and apply to area of the bite. Some little ones may have an allergic reaction to insect bites so it is important to keep an eye on the area for swelling or other signs of a reaction.

> **When to call a doctor**
>
> *Call a doctor if you notice anything abnormal about the bite. If your child suffers from an allergy, it is imperative that you seek immediate medical attention to assure that your child's health is not in danger. Call 911 or go directly to an ER if your child is suffering from shortness of breath, fever or an elevated heart rate.*

POISON IVY

Poison ivy is a poisonous plant that causes a rash when it comes into contact with human skin. Since it is very common, sometimes a baby can unknowingly come into contact with the plant. The poison can also be transferred from person to person, so if you, or someone you know, has poison ivy you should probably stay clear of handling baby.

How to Treat

If your little one has the unfortunate experience of contracting a poison ivy rash, there are a couple of things that you can do to help make them feel more comfortable. For little ones under the age of 6 months, it is important to get a doctor's recommendation on treatment. He will probably recommend that you bath your little one in an oatmeal bath using lukewarm water. Oatmeal is a classic skin treatment that helps alleviate all of the itching. Calamine lotion will also help alleviate the itching, this can be applied several times a day. Topical hydrocortisone cream and an oral antihistamine are other ways to treat itching, but make sure to speak to your doctor first.

When to call a doctor

You should see your doctor anytime your baby under 3 months contracts a rash, but if your baby is older, be sure to contact the doctor is the rash is accompanied by a fever. Signs of infection such as oozing or severe swelling are also grounds to contact your doctor. If baby's rash is keeping them awake at night or the rash has reached baby's face, it is important to seek medical attention.

FROSTBITE

Frostbite occurs when the skin is exposed to the extreme cold for too long a period of time. Since babies' skin is ultra-sensitive, this could happen very quickly. The first signs of frostbite are redness on the skin, but then it can progress to looking a yellowish color. Even if baby is bundled, frostbite can happen if any skin is exposed. It is usually seen on fingers, toes, and cheeks in babies, the areas that tend to be left uncovered or are easily exposed.

How to Treat

If your child is showing signs of frostbite, call the doctor or take him to your local ER. While on your way to get medical attention, stay calm and reassure baby that everything is going to be alright. If necessary, remove clothes and replace with new warmer clothes. Additionally, you should wrap baby in a warm blanket. Hold the areas affected in your hands to try and get them warm. Provide your baby with something warm to drink to help increase internal body temperature. If blisters have begun to form, do not touch them, instead, gently wrap gauze around fingers or toes that are affected to prevent further damage.

When to call a doctor

You should seek medical attention at the first signs of frostbite. Because frostbite takes place under the skin, often times there is more damage than what you actually see. Your doctor or emergency room staff will effectively treat your baby.

SUNBURN

Sunburn is exactly what is sounds like- burn from the sun. The first stages of sunburn look like reddened skin, but can later evolve into a darker, even purple color, and blisters on the skin. Sunburn can occur not only on babies' exposed skin, but also on skin that is covered by clothing. The sun is a super powerful orb that can penetrate clothing and cause the skin to be burned. Be sure to protect baby from sun by keeping them out of it entirely for the first 6 months of life.

How to Treat

The first thing that you should do at the sign of sunburn is remove baby from the sun. Get into a shaded area or go indoors. If either are available, cover baby with a towel or blanket to prevent further damage. Sunburn is extremely uncomfortable so it is important that you relieve baby's discomfort as much as possible. Keep baby hydrated, this will help them to fight off any infection the sunburn may cause. Offer baby as liquids more often than usual and possibly supplement with a baby electrolyte. Try a cool bath or cool cloth on the infected area for about 15 minutes at a time, and moisturize baby with an alcohol free lotion.

When to call a doctor

You should see a doctor if your baby is under a year old and has gotten sunburn. For all children, call a doctor if you notice the skin begin to blister, or if your child shows signs of swelling. It is also important to seek medical attention if there is any sign of infection or if your baby has a fever.

HEATSTROKE

Heatstroke is pretty serious business. Heatstroke is when the body's temperature gets too high, and the body cannot get the temperature down. It is caused when baby gets too hot and becomes overheated. If your child has a temperature above 103, he probably is suffering from heatstroke. This can happen from spending too much time outside in hot weather or being left in a hot car. Heatstroke usually starts off with signs of exhaustion or extreme thirst. If you notice that your baby is unusually thirsty and their skin is cool and moist, you may want to start treating for heatstroke.

How to Treat

If you suspect that your child is suffering from heatstroke, you need to call 911 right away. Time is of the essence in this situation so you will need to seek medical attention immediately. However, you must also take steps while waiting for help. If you are in the sun, get out of it. Find a shady area or a building with air conditioning. Also, get your hands on some cool water, sponge baby with a cloth or whatever you have on hand, and fan him to try and bring his external temperature down. If you can, bathe baby in cool water while you are waiting for an ambulance.

When to call a doctor?

Heatstroke is extremely dangerous. At the first signs of heatstroke, elevated heart rate, cool moist skin, flushed cheeks, exhaustion, extreme thirst, vomiting and rapid-

shallow breathing, call 911 and get to a medical professional immediately.

HEAT EXHAUSTION

Heat exhaustion takes place when your child's body temperature rises above normal body temperature. Signs of heat exhaustion are clammy skin, beat red color, or super pale, dizziness or fainting. His heart rate may seem to be higher than normal and he may appear to be very thirsty.

How to Treat

If you are noticing any of these symptoms, get baby out of heat source. It is important to try to lower body temperature as soon as possible. If you are directly in the sun, go into the shade or an air conditioned area if possible. Try to get baby to take in some fluids like water or a drink containing electrolytes. Loosen or remove clothing and fan down baby's skin to try and lower body temperature. If you can, cool down baby with a cold cloth and fan with a magazine or portable fan if you have one.

When to call a doctor

You should seek medical attention if you cannot get baby back to normal body temperature within an hour. If you see more severe symptoms like loss of consciousness or an inability to breathe, take him to the ER right away.

ALLERGY

An allergy is simply an immune response to an external allergen. Baby's response to an allergen can range from a reaction that results in a rash, cough, runny nose, sneezing or itching. Or the reaction may be more severe such as one that causes anaphylactic shock.

How to Treat

Your best bet is to get a doctor's diagnosis before treating an allergy. In order to properly treat, it is important to know exactly what you are treating. A doctor can administer tests that will determine what your baby is allergic to and guide you towards treatment that will try and alleviate symptoms. Because allergies are a reaction to an external source, if your baby is allergic to, let's say dust mites, it would be important to change and launder sheets regularly and possibly implement the use of an air purifier in the home. Once your baby is diagnosed with a specific allergy, follow the recommendations of your medical professional on how to treat it.

When to call a doctor

You should take your baby to the ER immediately if you notice that your baby is having difficulty breathing or is unconscious. You should make an appointment with your doctor any time you see a reaction that is unusual.

DIABETIC EMERGENCY

A diabetic emergency occurs when there is a severe drop in insulin. This can send your little one into shock, and the experience can be haunting. Sometimes diabetic emergencies present themselves with your child fainting, or you may find that your child becomes disengaged with reality, unable to form words or make eye contact.

How to Treat

In order to effectively treat a diabetic emergency, which can come on suddenly and unexpected, you should be well trained. If you are not, you should call 911 immediately and try to stay calm while you are waiting for the responders to arrive. If you have the equipment, check the child's blood sugar. In the meantime try to give the child some juice or a lollipop to try to bring them out of shock. If the child is unconscious or unresponsive, be sure that they are positioned on their side, in a safe space, free from being able to cause injury or harm to themselves if they begin to convulse. Call 911 and stay with the child until help arrives.

> **When to call a doctor**
>
> *Call 911 or seek immediate medical attention at the first signs of a diabetic emergency.*

FAINTING

Fainting is the sudden loss of total consciousness. It is more than just falling asleep, but a more immediate reaction. Your child could be vividly alert one second and in an instant lose all alertness and muscle control.

How to Treat

If your child faints, first check and be sure that he is still breathing. Once you have established that, try to lean him forward with his head in between his knees. Your child may be dehydrated or improperly nourished, so make sure to offer them something to drink as soon as they are alert. Because fainting is not common in younger children, it is advised that you seek medical attention as soon as possible to determine the cause of the fainting.

When to call a doctor

If your child is not breathing or you do not feel like your child is acting right, it is best to take him to the emergency room right away. If your child fainted after a bump to the head or serious fall, getting immediate medical attention is the best thing to do.

FEVER

A fever is defined as a temperature above 100.4 degrees. It is usually accompanied with reddish cheeks and skin radiating heat. The classic way to test for a fever is to feel baby's forehead with the back of your hand, if it feels more hot than normal, you should take his temperature with a thermometer. Although rectal temperatures are most accurate, any thermometer will give you a sign if baby has a fever.

How to Treat

To treat fever, first keep baby hydrated. If he seems uncomfortable or fussy, you may want to administer a fever reducer such as ibuprofen or acetaminophen. Be sure to get your doctor's advice first. Also, let baby sleep. If baby is sleeping longer than usual, it might be a sign that his body is taking the time to fight off the infection or whatever is causing the fever. Just keep the environment cool, and baby comfortable in loose fitting clothes. If possible, keep baby in just his diaper and cover him with a loose blanket. A cool bath can also help alleviate discomfort, or you can give baby a sponge bath, wiping him down with a cool cloth several times a day.

When to call a doctor

You should seek immediate medical attention if your baby is under 3 months. Infants do not show the same signs of infection of older children. Also, if a child's fever is exceptionally high. A fever above 104 can be dangerous and warrants at least a phone call to ask if you should take further action. Otherwise, if other symptoms are present with the fever like vomiting, shaking, or fainting, you should go see a doctor. If a fever lasts more than 24 hours, and over-the counter medicines are not helping, call and get medical advice.

EPILEPTIC SEIZURE

Seizures in babies can range in type and intensity. Some seizures may cause parts of baby's body to stiffen, while others may appear as baby's head to be nodding. Another type of seizure will cause baby to stop all motions and only their eyes will move from side to side.

How to Treat

Epileptic seizure requires the medical attention and diagnosis of a professional. If you suspect that your baby is having an epileptic seizure, it is important that you get him to a doctor right away. Because of the range of types of seizures there is not one way to treat them. Once diagnosed, treatment will most likely come in the form of a prescribed medicine. Your doctor can then give you the proper protocol to take if these situations ever arise again.

When to see a doctor

Take baby to doctor or Emergency Room as soon as you suspect that he is having an epileptic episode.

EARACHE

An earache occurs when baby is exhibiting that he has pain coming from his ear. There can be several causes for an earache, but most commonly it is due to an infection. Baby can also get an earache from having an object or water stuck in his ear.

How to Treat

It is important to first assess the situation. Figure out if the pain is coming from a physical object in baby's ear. If not, you can ease the pain of the earache by providing baby with ibuprofen or acetaminophen, just be sure to check with your doctor first for proper dosing. You can also try to ease pain with a warm cloth near the ear, but not in it. You should always see a doctor if your child is suffering from any ear pain.

When to see a doctor

Earaches are usually signs that there is something wrong. If your child seems to be suffering from ear pain call a doctor right away. They may have an ear infection, or something may have entered the ear causing your baby to become uncomfortable, both which should be treated by a medical professional.

TOOTHACHE

A toothache occurs when baby feels pain at the sight of a tooth. This can be due to teething if your baby has not yet received any teeth. If your child has teeth already, a toothache can be the result of a cavity, or blunt force to a tooth.

How to treat

If your child is suffering from tooth pain, it is important to call a dentist right away. Pain usually implies that there is another underlying issue that needs to be resolved.

[2]

COMMON INFANT ILLNESSES

A SICK BABY IS never any fun! But how do you know when you should be worried? This is your baby you are talking about—you should always be worried! But not all illness are alike. This section covers some of the most common infant illnesses and what are signs you need to call the doctor.

COMMON COLD

Due to the immaturity of baby's immune system, it is more than likely that he will get more than a few in his first few years of life. Due to the numerous amount of germs and viruses that cause the common cold, it is hard to pinpoint exactly what a cold looks like. Your baby may have a cough or a runny nose with clear mucous that turns to a yellow or green over time. He may also become congested and contract a low grade fever.

There is really nothing to do if your child has a cold except keep them hydrated with lots of fluids. Because colds come from a variety of viruses, unfortunately it just has to run its course. Rest, relaxation and chicken soup is the best combination for your toddler if he comes down with the common cold. For infants, you may want to try to offer them more feedings to keep them ultra hydrated. To ease the uncomfortable side effects of a cold, a humidifier can help with congestion. Alternatively, you can run the hot shower and bring baby into the bathroom for a bit. For the unfortunate constant mucus in the nose, saline and suction are a good combination. If your infant is to get a cold, make sure to keep an eye on him. A fever may be a sign of a more serious illness and you should take them to the doctor right away.

Since colds are pretty common, once your little one gets one, you will be familiar with treatment. However, it is important to take infants under three months to the doctor if you feel that they are sick, especially if they have a temperature over 100 degrees. If your baby is over 2 and has a fever for over 24 hours, it's time to go to the doctor. Also, if your baby has a cough that lasts longer than a week, you should seek medical attention. If you feel that you are unsure that baby has a cold or something worse, go with your gut. It won't hurt to get doctor's opinion on what is wrong and how to treat baby effectively.

INFLUENZA

Influenza or the Flu is a serious disease. If not treated immediately it can cause major complications, even death. Be sure that if you notice signs of the flu in baby you take him to the doctor immediately. Babies who have the flu may seem extremely lethargic. Also, they may have a cough that just doesn't seem to go away. The flu can also cause baby to have trouble breathing, or change baby's skin tone to a bluish color. Fever is usually prominent, and baby may not want to interact at all.

If you suspect that baby may have Influenza, you must get him to the doctor right away. The flu can cause a number of problems, including dehydration. For young children, especially infants, dehydration can be detrimental to health. Because the flu is viral, there is little that can be done, however, a doctor will most likely administer an antiviral to try and speed the healing process up. In the meantime, it is important to keep baby hydrated, offering them more than normal feedings or drinks. Since he probably won't feel good enough to eat, offer baby small meals or snacks. If baby has a high fever, cool them down with a moist cloth or in a cool tub. If advised by the doctor, you may administer ibuprofen or acetaminophen if you feel your baby is uncomfortable due to fever or other symptoms.

COLD

VERSUS

FLU

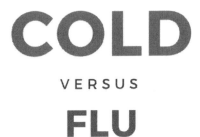

FLU	COLD
Symtoms Abrupt	Symtoms Gradual
Fever Common	Fever Uncommon
Sneezing Uncommon	Sneezing Common
Sore Throat Uncommon	Sore Throat Common

RSV

RSV is less commonly referred to as Respiratory syncytial virus. It is a common respiratory virus that resembles the common cold in children and adults, but could be very dangerous, even life threatening in babies 2 and under. The virus is spread through the air or through contact. Baby can get RSV from being near a sneeze of someone with RSV or from person to person contact with someone who has the virus.

If you notice that your little one is suffering from symptoms such as runny nose, cough, poor appetite, irritability and wheezing or rapid breathing, he may have RSV. You should get medical attention right away to ensure that you take the right steps towards getting baby back to being better. RSV can lead to bigger and more dangerous conditions so the sooner you see the doctor the better. Because it is viral in nature, there is no real cure for RSV. Like every other virus, RSV will have to run its course. You can help the process more comfortable by offering your child lots of liquids, use a cool mist vaporizer to help with congestion, and use saline to help break up mucus. Do not use over the counter medications unless you get the okay from your doctor first.

If your baby has symptoms of RSV, it is important to get them to the doctor. RSV has been known to cause more serious conditions like pneumonia and bronchiolitis, both of which are serious lung disorders that require immediate attention. If your baby has common cold symptoms in addition to blue/grey skin, extreme fatigue, and high fever, it is important to see a doctor right away.

ROSEOLA

Roseola, also known as sixth disease, is a very contagious virus that is easily spread from person to person through saliva or respiratory droplets, like sneezing. It is caused by a strain of the herpes virus, but it is not the same as the sexually transmitted disease. It is most common among children between the ages of 3 months and 4 years of age and is accompanied by a high fever and a pink rash that starts in the middle and extends to the limbs.

There is no real treatment for Roseola as it is viral in nature. Unfortunately, it will just have to run its course. However, there are some things that you can do to try and make the process less painful for baby. First off, keep baby hydrated. Give them plenty of fluids throughout the day. Offer more feedings, or supplement with an infant electrolyte drink. To try and keep fever down, give baby lukewarm baths, and let them air dry instead of toweling off. Furthermore, keep them in loose fitted clothing, or just a diaper if weather and temperature permit. You may be able to give baby acetaminophen, but check with doctor first.

Any time your baby has a rash and a fever, you should call a doctor. Although it is viral, it is important to have doctor take a look to make sure it has not progressed into something else.

GASTROENTERITIS

Gastroenteritis is a bowel infection, usually viral, that causes baby to have diarrhea. Sometimes vomiting can also occur. It is common in babies and young children, especially those who go to daycare. It is easily spread through contact, so it is very important to wash hands regularly to prevent the spread of the virus. There are different strains of the virus, so it is possible that baby can contract gastroenteritis more than once.

Since your baby will probably not want to eat anything during a bout with gastroenteritis, it is extremely important to keep them hydrated. Providing more than usual opportunities is imperative in order to prevent dehydration. Signs of dehydration include dry mouth, sunken eyes, unusual sleepiness, and cold hands and feet. Check diapers to make sure baby is passing urine, no wet diapers are a sign of dehydration. Because it is common for diarrhea to last up to ten days, you want to be sure to keep baby clean. Be sure to check diaper frequently not only to see if changes are necessary, but to make sure a rash has not taken over. Diarrhea can cause severe diaper rash, so you should have some diaper ointment on hand to help alleviate any pain on baby's bottom.

You should see a doctor if your baby is less than 3 months and has a fever over 10 degrees. It is also important that you seek medical attention if you notice any signs of dehydration. Younger babies tend to dehydrate quicker and this can cause serious complications. Make sure that if your baby is super lethargic and difficult to wake that you go to the doctor. If you see blood in the stool or vomit, it is imperative that you see the doctor right away. If there is anything that makes you uncomfortable or worried about baby, you should seek medical attention.

HAND FOOT AND MOUTH DISEASE

Hand Foot and Mouth Disease is a common viral illness that can affect little ones. It is more common for children up to age 5, but can also be found in older children. Typical symptoms of Hand Foot and Mouth disease is a rash on the palms of hands and soles of feet, and blisters may also form. Sometimes rashes can form in other areas such as the genital area, buttocks, knees or elbows. Children may also complain of a sore throat and become tired and dehydrated as a result of this disease.

If you suspect that your child has Hand Foot and Mouth Disease, you should make an appointment to see your doctor right away. Even though it is viral and has to run its course, you want to be sure to get the proper diagnosis and the proper treatment. As all viral infections, Hand Foot and Mouth Disease will have no particular treatment, but there are things that you can do to alleviate symptoms. Since sores may form in the mouth, and numbing mouthwash may be recommended by your doctor, however, do not administer without the proper guidance. Make sure to keep other family members safe by washing hands frequently, and there should be no physical contact such as hugging or kissing. Keep your little one hydrated with fluids, and for babies still breastfeeding or drinking bottles, be sure to offer more frequent feedings.

FIFTH'S DISEASE

Fifth's disease is another common childhood disease that is scarier than it sounds. It is a common illness that is caused by the parvovirus and is easily recognizable by the bright, red circles that form on your child's cheeks. Fifth's disease may also reveal itself through cold-like symptoms like runny nose, sore throat and muscles, fever, and fatigue. Although it is not dangerous for your little one, it can be dangerous for pregnant women as the disease can pass from mom to fetus.

As with other viral treatments, Fifth's Disease does not have a specific course of action. Since it has to run its course, Fifth's Disease can only be treated symptomatically. You can do certain things to make your baby more comfortable, but you will have to wait it out for symptoms to subside. One thing you can do is keep your child hydrated and give them oatmeal baths to alleviate symptoms. Under the direction of a doctor, you may also want to administer pain relieving medications like ibuprofen or acetaminophen. Oral antihistamines may also be recommended, but check with your doctor first for proper dosing. Make sure you keep your doctor informed if your child starts to develop more serious symptoms such as swelling or high fevers. If you are pregnant and have been exposed to Fifth's Disease, it is extremely important that you notify your doctor right away so he can advise you on the proper steps to take to keep you and your baby healthy.

STREP THROAT

Strep throat is caused by Streptococcus bacteria that initiates a variety of symptoms. It will be hard to tell if baby has strep throat for sure without a doctor's diagnosis, but there are some sure tell signs. For one, baby's tonsils will be enlarged and swollen. A fever may also accompany the infection, along with a headache, stomach ache, and sometimes vomiting. In some cases, baby may contract a rash all over his body, which is also referred to as Scarlet Fever.

In order to treat strep, it is important to first get a diagnosis. Because strep is a bacterial infection, antibiotics will be administered. A conversation with your pediatrician is a must to ensure that the antibiotics are not going to cause an allergic reaction. Other things that you can do to alleviate the discomforts of strep are to provide lots and lots of liquids for baby. Staying hydrated is key for any infection. Since a sore throat usually accompanies strep, cold ice pops or drinks may help ease the pain in the throat. You may also give your child ibuprofen or acetaminophen, but speak to your doctor first for correct dosing. Strep is severely contagious so the sooner you see a doctor the better. Make sure to switch toothbrushes and bedsheets after you start the antibiotic to prevent a relapse.

You should definitely see a doctor as soon as you suspect that baby may have strep. Since it is bacterial a prescription will be needed to cure the sickness. The sooner you see a doctor, the sooner baby will feel better.

PINKEYE

If your baby starts to show signs of mildly red eyelids and some tearing, he may have contracted pinkeye. Pink Eye or conjunctivitis is inflammation of baby's eye. This can be caused by an irritant, bacteria or a virus, and the latter two are very contagious. Pink Eye becomes obvious when the whites of baby's eyes become red, the lower or upper eyelids are inflamed, and there is goop or puss oozing from the eye.

If you notice signs of pink eye, it is very important to contact your pediatrician. Treatment will be determined by doctor, depending on the strain. If it is viral, there is really nothing you can do. A warm compress on the eye may be comforting, however, you will have to wait for the strain to takes its course. If the strain is bacterial, your doctor will most likely prescribe an antibiotic drop that will clear up the infection quickly and painlessly. For both cases, doctor will most likely recommend a warm compress and suggest that you wipe away dried discharge to keep baby comfortable.

PINWORMS

Although they can be upsetting to parents, pinworms are a common childhood ailment. Especially among those who go to daycare or have siblings that are school age. Pinworms are tiny, string-like worms that invade the intestines. They can cause itching and irritation around the anus, causing your baby to become very uncomfortable. Pinworms are easily transferable. Your child can pick them up simply by using a toy that was previously used by someone who was infected. The worms end up in the mouth and travel to the intestine where the female will lay eggs, and the cycle will continue from there.

In order to treat pinworms, you should take your child to the doctor. Your doctor will probably prescribe medication for baby, and the whole family, to ensure that anyone who was carrying worms can eliminate them from their system, since they are so easily transferred from one person to the next. The doctor may suggest that a second round of treatment is implemented a few weeks later to ensure that all pinworms have been eliminated from everyone's system. Prevention is key when it comes to an ailment like pinworms. Be sure to keep hands clean and change bedding after infestation occurs.

BOOKS IN
THE RIDICULOUSLY SIMPLE PARENTING
SERIES

The Ridiculously Simple Guide to Baby First Aide

The Ridiculously Simple Guide to Breastfeeding

The Ridiculously Simple Guide to Cesarean Section

The Ridiculously Simple Guide Cloth Diapering

The Ridiculously Simple Guide to Co-Sleeping

The Ridiculously Simple Guide to Postpartum

The Ridiculously Simple Guide to Teething

The Ridiculously Simple Guide to Sleep Training

ABOUT THE AUTHOR

Margo Jean is a freelance writer and the mother of a son and daughter (both clothed diapered, of course!). When she's not writing or watching her kids, you can find her shooting photos with one of her many vintage cameras.

Printed in Great Britain
by Amazon